BIOMAGNETISM HEALING

Will it work for you?

A book of hope by Rosemary Walters

Biomagnetism Healing: Will it Work for You?

Copyright © 2024 Rosemary Walters

Published by Disruptive Publishing

www.disruptivepublishing.com.au

As told to Rhonda Valentine Dixon

Edited by Rhonda Valentine Dixon

Photography by Katie Bennett www.embellysh.com.au

All Rights Reserved. No part of this publication may be reproduced, distributed or transmitted in any form, or by any means, including photocopying, recording, or any other electronic methods, without the prior written permission of the author or publisher. Brief quotations that are credited to the publication and the author are permitted.

978-1-7637283-3-2 Kindle
978-1-7637283-2-5 Print

Disclaimers

AI Disclaimer

No part of this publication may be reproduced, stored or used in any form or by any means, including but not limited to artificial intelligence systems, machine learning models, or automated data processing technologies, for training analysis, or any other purpose, without the prior written permission of the copyright holder. This work is protected by copyright law, and unauthorized use by AI or related technologies is strictly prohibited.

Disclaimer

The information presented in this book regarding biomagnetism is intended for informational and educational purposes only. Biomagnetism, as discussed herein, is an alternative or complementary health practice that involves the application of magnets to specific areas of the body with the intention of promoting wellness. However, readers should be aware of several important considerations before engaging with or relying on this practice.

Biomagnetism Does Not Work for Everyone

The effects of biomagnetism vary widely. While some people may report perceived benefits from the use of this discipline, there is no guarantee it will produce similar results for all individuals. Factors such as health conditions, physiological differences, and other variables, may influence outcomes. The efficacy of biomagnetism has not been universally established and it may not be effective for every person or every condition. Readers are encouraged to approach biomagnetism with open-mindedness. The writers also acknowledge the wisdom of consulting with a qualified healthcare professional before using it as part of an established health regimen.

Anecdotal Nature of Examples

The examples, testimonials, and case studies included in this book are anecdotal in nature and reflect the personal experiences of specific individuals. These accounts are not intended to represent typical or expected results for all users of biomagnetism. The experiences described are subjective and may not be replicable. They are included to illustrate how some individuals have engaged with biomagnetism, not as evidence of guaranteed or widespread outcomes. Readers should not assume that their experience with biomagnetism will mirror the examples provided in this book.

Lack of Peer-Reviewed Scientific Studies

To date, there are no peer-reviewed scientific studies available that conclusively validate the efficacy or mechanisms of biomagnetism as a therapeutic practice. While some proponents of biomagnetism suggest that it may influence bodily processes, these claims have not been substantiated through rigorous, controlled scientific research published in reputable, peer-reviewed journals. The absence of such studies means that biomagnetism remains an experimental and unproven approach in the context of evidence-based medicine. Readers should use critical judgement when considering biomagnetism, particularly in the absence of robust scientific evidence.

Hypothetical Nature of Localised pH Alteration

One of the proposed mechanisms of biomagnetism involves the alteration of localised pH levels in the body to promote health or address imbalances. This concept is, at this stage, a hypothesis and has not been empirically validated through scientific research. The idea that applying magnets to specific areas of the body can meaningfully alter localised pH levels, and that such changes result in therapeutic benefits, remains speculative. Without peer-reviewed studies to support this hypothesis, it should not be regarded as a proven mechanism of action. Readers are advised to approach this and other theoretical claims about biomagnetism judiciously and to seek whether it is complementary to treatments prescribed by qualified medical professionals.

General Health and Safety Considerations

Biomagnetism is not a substitute for conventional medical diagnosis, treatment, or care. It should not be used to replace professional medical advice or interventions prescribed by licensed healthcare providers. Individuals with medical conditions, those who are pregnant, or those with implanted medical devices (such as pacemakers or insulin pumps) should consult a healthcare professional before attempting biomagnetism, as magnets may interfere with certain medical devices or conditions. This book does not provide medical advice, and readers should not rely on its contents to diagnose, treat, cure or prevent any disease or health condition.

Responsibility of the Reader

The decision to explore or practice biomagnetism is solely the responsibility of the reader. The authors, publishers and contributors to this book make no warranties, express or implied, regarding the safety, efficacy, or suitability of biomagnetism for any individual or purpose. By choosing to engage with biomagnetism, readers assume all risks associated with its use. The authors and publishers disclaim any liability for adverse effects, losses, or damages that may arise from the application of the information presented in this book.

Consultation with Healthcare Professionals

We strongly recommend that readers consult with a licensed healthcare provider before incorporating biomagnetism into their health practices. This is particularly important for individuals with pre-existing medical conditions, those taking medications, or those seeking treatment for specific health concerns. A qualified healthcare professional can provide personalised guidance regarding ensuring that any complementary practices, including biomagnetism, are safe and appropriate for the patient's individual circumstances.

By reading this book, you acknowledge that you have read and understood this disclaimer and agree to use the information provided at your own discretion and risk.

.

Dedication

This book is dedicated to Lisa Brough.

Lisa, your unwavering dedication and tireless efforts to expand the reach and availability of biomagnetism to Australians have not gone unnoticed.

Through your commitment, passion and perseverance, countless lives have been touched, and a once lesser-known field of holistic health is now more accessible to those in need. Your work has laid the foundation for a healthier and more balanced future for many.

Thank you for your vision, your hard work, and your steadfast belief in the power of biomagnetism. You are truly an inspiration to us all.

Table of Contents

Foreword..13

Introduction..15

PART I MY STORY...17

Chapter One: Growing Up 19

Chapter Two: Leaving Home 29

Chapter Three: Settling Down................................41

Chapter Four: Finding a Lump...............................51

Chapter Five: Finding Biomagnetism....................57

PART II MAGNETS AND HEALING 65

PART III STORIES OF SUCCESS...................................91

Praise for Rosemary Walters and for Biomagnetism Healing..93

Susan's Story...96

Rhonda's Story..98

Lisa Pearson's Story *100*

Lisa Brough's Story *102*

Minnie's Story *107*

Patricia's Story *108*

Work with Rosemary *111*

Acknowledgments *115*

Further Reading *119*

A note from Rhonda Valentine Dixon *125*

Foreword

I clearly remember meeting Rosemary for the first time. I was hosting our local Spiritual Meet-up group at my home. Her warmth, intelligence and genuine nature drew me in instantly. Where we often take a while to size someone up, I could tell right away she was a bright, caring soul with her feet firmly planted on the ground.

Shortly after, she confided in me about her health concern.

You may wonder how someone so full of light came to have such health challenges.

But as all of us come to discover at some point... the human experience is complex. The mind/body/spirit connections are real and convoluted. Together she and I explored the factors that led to her health breaking down—the mundane physical reasons, the emotional, self-esteem, spiritual and relationship themes.

Rosemary's openness, humility, curiosity and willingness to heal have served her well as she moved through her health issues. There has been immense learning and growth.

Her life story is one many Australian women can relate to, in particular country women. It's the sort of life centred in caring, relationships and hard work. And how you show up when you are meeting life's challenges. You bring all your energy, values, experience and willingness to the task.

Her family is blessed to have her.

We, her friends and colleagues, are lucky to know her.

In a world where most people think caring is a feeling within their chest, Rosemary is a shining example of the meaning of caring through doing. She is the first to offer "what can I do to help?" And we are so grateful she has made the move to become a facilitator of healing with Biomagnetism to serve others.

"What can I do to help?" with Magnets in hand.

~ *Lisa Brough. Holistic Biomagnetist and Mentor*

Introduction

Dear Friend,

Perhaps you're wondering how you got to this point of 'unwellness'. Maybe it crept up, a pathogenic infection, maybe a genetic issue or some other explanation has been offered for your condition, or no explanation at all, but it just doesn't feel like you should be struggling as much as you are each day.

I have been where you are. It can be confusing and sometimes it can be quite scary.

Illnesses can take their mental and emotional toll and when we feel stressed, we are compromising our body's healing ability, so it turns into a very unhelpful cycle, and you may begin to wonder if anything will work for you.

If this sounds like you, know that you are not alone, and that there are things that will help.

When I was at this point with my own health, I had tried other treatments, researched online, and been to several health professionals without finding anything that offered much genuine or lasting healing. Then I found biomagnetism.

For me, it was life changing. And now, here I am writing a book about it so that I can help you negotiate whatever you are going through.

By the time you find biomagnetism, you may have all but given up hope and you might feel like you need a miracle.

I see you. I hear you. I know what a difference magnets made for me and now I want to help you, so please, read on.

Let's find out if biomagnetism will work for you and change your life the way it changed mine. What have you got to lose?

Warm regards,

Rosemary

Love, Light and Healing

PART I

MY STORY

Chapter One: Growing Up

In the Beginning

My first meaningful conversations with my father occurred in our yard. Dad delighted in showing me the enchanting realm that was our garden. I would follow him around and listen to him talk about the flora. He'd name each plant and spell out both the generic and botanical names. To this day he talks to us about what grows in our gardens.

As a child, my sister Elise wasn't in the slightest bit interested in Dad's garden. But she fell in love with plants in adulthood and committed to memory many botanical names. Though she may not be aware of it, having memorised so much is an endearing way of showing our father she now shares his love of nature. And he, by the simple gesture of sharing his knowledge of the garden with us as children, was developing caring communication which endures to this day.

Our mother, a microbiologist, was as at ease telling us about the chemical chain of events that occur when alcohol breaks down in the body (and such things) as she was being the mum who did all the daily parenting tasks a mother does.

With scientists for parents, it was likely we'd be introduced to intelligent discourse early. The above descriptions of my parents exemplify this. As a child I didn't know how fortunate I was, but I'm glad of it now. My parents' stories provided a wonderful grounding for learning and fostered a trusting bond between parent and child. And their open-mindedness was the example I needed to inspire me to come to the place I am at present.

My father worked as an apiary officer. He had a passion for nature and a dedication to bees. An apiarist *must* understand the ecological system to ensure the biosecurity of bees and to maximise quality honey production.

Despite easy displays of his deep passion for his work Dad did not, with the same ease, give physical demonstrations of affection to his children (two boys and

Chapter One:
Growing Up

two girls). Rather than being showered with hugs and kisses, he shared with us, with a caring heart, his vast knowledge of nature.

Mum wasn't a hugger either. Her love for us manifested in her motherly duties. The fruits of her labour were consistently evident in the cake tins. Delicious homemade cakes, and biscuits complemented the sandwiches and fresh fruit in our school lunch boxes. She drove us to school on rainy days, and she provided nutritious meals, though we ate with decorum. The dinner table wasn't the place for animated discussion. Mother would have liked more conversation, but our father insisted mealtimes were for practicing table manners.

To this day the intelligence and worldly wisdom in both parents is still acutely clear. They continue to be discerning in their choices, discuss topics openly and question with genuine interest.

Mum, Dad and Travel

In their younger days, Mum and Dad explored the world extensively. Our intrepid mother travelled alone on a boat to Argentina and worked for a year as a nanny in Buenos Aires. She learned Spanish from the children she cared for. Her free time was spent in the Teatro Colón where she heard and absorbed the language in the operas presented there. For the equivalent of twenty cents, Mum could stand 'with the Gods' in the theatre's highest points. There she would be totally immersed in the voices of international artists like Enrico Caruso and Maria Callas, transmitted by the theatre's exceptional acoustics.

Mum lived and worked in London for about a year, too. London was (and still is) a must for a young traveller, especially if they enjoy cultural pursuits.

Much later, when we children were approaching our teens, Mum returned to study and achieved a botany degree.

Dad also lived and worked in London for a while. He was an inspector of Australian fruit. He was employed to check the quality of imported fruits and vegetables, both in the capital and in other English and continental ports when the need for his expertise arose.

Chapter One:
Growing Up

I don't doubt my parents' experiences and travels fostered the care they have for others, in addition to strengthening their global mindset.

Lately, their time is spent in favoured pleasurable pursuits, such as a book club, Tai Chi, Mahjong, craft and handiwork for Mum, and gardening and photography for Dad. They also share a love for travelling.

Family Life

As a child, I enjoyed my parents' stories and our family discussions. All the interaction was enlightening and confirmed for me that intelligence was a worthy attribute to have. The topics our parents introduced us to may not have been the norm in every local household, but other aspects of my childhood were typical of our community.

We lived in Warwick, a small town where it was safe to ride our bikes the 1.5 km uphill journey to primary school. Then, with the school day over, we delighted in the thrill of a swift downhill ride home.

High school was further away, but we walked because it we considered it 'uncool' to ride our bikes. We knew people along the way, so there was little concern for our safety. Mum and Dad were much more perturbed if we forgot to 'slop on sunscreen' or 'slap on our hats' (or helmets when we rode).

Neighbourhood kids played in their yard (or someone else's) most afternoons and weekends. The benefits of this, our health and fitness, didn't occur to us then, but we were healthier of mind and body, than some children are now, with today's easy access to fast food and sedentary pastimes.

With only one class per year level, our primary school was small. I fell naturally into the role of a good student who followed the rules. Though I was eager to 'have a go' at most things, for no apparent reason, I felt apart from the other students.

In early high school, my perception was that I would be more comfortable in the 'smart people' cohort, so that's where I gravitated to. That feeling of not having a lot in common with others has stayed with me well into adulthood, but maturity ensures I cope with it better. I am more at ease with accepting me for who I am now.

Chapter One:
Growing Up

I was a reasonably sporty child, which was just as well because television only presented one, (and later, two) channels. My parents were discerning about *everything*, including the programmes their children viewed. I can remember watching *Play School* and *Sesame Street* and a couple of innocuous cartoons, *Roger Ramjet* and *Inspector Gadget*. Each protagonist in the latter two, was a likeable though dim-witted hero saving the world in every episode. But, in our parents' eyes, more important to watch because we learned from them, were David Attenborough documentaries. Everybody knew Attenborough's work and some of my friends were also brought up on his documentaries.

I made friends at school but preferred to spend my time with one close friend at a time. Over the years, I have been fortunate to have been enriched by relationships with a few close friends, not necessarily all at the same time. Women need other women. Communication with trusted friends is our way of seeking to unravel life's conundrums and mysteries and make sense of our world. I love having special friends I can talk to about anything. But conversely, I have always enjoyed and hope to continue to enjoy a bunch of friends on the periphery as well.

As a child I was interested in healing and I considered being a doctor, however the amount of study and training involved was daunting, so that idea didn't become a desire. At thirteen, I knew what I wanted to be. A music teacher. My self-discipline regarding schoolwork and music practice was paying off. I had a goal now and was determined to work towards it.

With three teenagers, one child still at primary school and very busy parents, things could get a little stressful at home. Mum and I had some heated differences of opinion, as most teenagers do with their parents. The idea of sending me away to boarding school was broached. It was a good option for us all, not just because of those mother/daughter arguments, but because Mum, Dad and I all felt I needed more choices in my last years of school. So off I went to Toowoomba for years eleven and twelve.

Chapter One:
Growing Up

Boarding School

The possibility of boarding school could have rocked the confidence of some girls. They might have been apprehensive at the thought of leaving their family behind. And moving away from friends whose influence and company they, in their mid-teens, might have sought over that of parents and siblings, could also have been daunting. But none of that mattered to me. I was happy in my own company. Why wouldn't I be? I had purpose.

Together, my parents and I chose a Catholic boarding school. I'd grown up Anglican, but I practised neither faith, so any quality school was okay with me. We needed to consider the calibre of the education, greater subject choice, and a better music curriculum with a more experienced piano teacher over an adherence to a particular Christian doctrine.

So out into the world I went.

I became one of fifty-five boarders in a big old communal Queenslander in Toowoomba. This was one of three boarding houses at my school and there were students from years seven to twelve in attendance. I studied and practiced the piano by day and watched Pretty Woman and Top Gun on continual repeat in out-of-school hours. Of course I missed my family. I loved them, and they loved me, but overall my years at boarding school were happy.

Chapter Two: Leaving Home

Out Into the World I Go

Upon completing school, I applied for the Queensland University of Technology's four years, double bachelor's degree, music/education course. It was perfect for me. When I was accepted, I had my life planned out. I'd study, teach music, travel, perhaps live and work overseas, meet a special someone, get married, buy a house, and have children. Well, that was the plan, anyway.

While diligently executing my grand plan and training to teach music to high school students, I endured such a ghastly experience with the teens in my final practicum that I chose instead to focus on primary school children. The work experience I shared with the younger kids had been satisfying, and I could immediately see where my strengths lay.

I took a position in an Innisfail school (while also teaching piano privately outside school hours) and delighted in watching my students grow and revel in the joy music gave them. Watching the children emerge from uncertainty to accomplishment and seeing how they felt when they achieved well, particularly when they didn't think they could, gave me immense satisfaction. And I loved challenging my students, pushing them to stretch past what was comfortable and achieve beyond their own expectations.

Time to Fly

Though I enjoyed teaching classroom music, by age twenty-five I felt it was time for a change; to seek adventures beyond small-town far north Queensland. I applied and was granted a transfer from Innisfail to the Gold Coast, a region I thought would be vibrant and fun for a young teacher. Simultaneously, I applied to teach in the United Arab Emirates. I achieved both positions.

I requested leave from the Queensland Education Department and began to plan for another of my life goals—to live and work overseas. Once again, my

Chapter Two:
Leaving Home

parents gave me their carefully considered advice and their invaluable encouragement.

My initial posting was at the first International Australian School in Sharjah in the United Arab Emirates. I was thrilled to be accepted but was astounded when a friend expressed a particularly discouraging remark, 'You don't know what they hide under those burkas', she said.

I expect the comment was meant to ensure I was aware Muslims were unfamiliar, and I needed to be careful. But to me, it was a bizarre thing to say, and I felt it suggested the speaker was less worldly wise than I was accustomed to in people her age. A simple 'take care, Rosemary' would have sufficed if she really felt it necessary.

Besides, I was on a high. I was ready to tick off another exciting goal in my grand plan and I had the joy of music to share with children of different cultures. I loved the fact that the global knowledge of music was another form of communication. A language understood by all. As for the opinion expressed by my older friend, the notion that another nation's womenfolk might conceal upon their person an implement with which to do me harm hadn't even entered my head.

The United Arab Emirates

How much hotter could my new home be than far north Queensland? Disembarking the plane in Sharjah at 2.00 am in 37-degree heat was the promise of things to come. We were lucky if it rained two days a year in the UAE and a Queensland summer was akin to an Emirates spring. If walking from my car to the school buildings in over 40-degree heat in the morning was unpleasant, returning to the car in the afternoon was utterly ghastly. Sitting in my car after it had been in the sun all day was like being in an airless desert.

'Oh, but we *are* in the desert', I reminded myself. Well, hadn't I ticked off the 'live and teach overseas' goal in spectacular fashion?

The Australian International School—My First Posting

The Australian International School was in Industrial Area 18 in Sharjah, relatively close to Dubai. The school accessed the highest quality instruction in the

Chapter Two:
Leaving Home

Queensland school curriculum. It also offered modules in Arabic and Islamic Studies. There was a vibrancy about AIS which was reflected in its mission statement. The school sought to *'develop high-achieving, well-rounded students who were connected globally, to each other, and to the communities in which they would live and serve'*.[1]

Well, that was certainly a reasonable aim. And it started right there in the classroom. I was presented with multiple nationalities of children in my class, who would foster friendships as children do. Since they all came from high achieving parents who were the designers, engineers, and builders of the infrastructure of this extraordinary place there was a reasonable likelihood these children would one day accomplish whatever they dreamed of in their own communities and beyond.

The school's vision was to *'provide a quality international and intercultural education that prepared the students for working in a global economy'*.[2] Learning English was a part

---

[1] Australian International School, https://www.ais.ae/about-us/vision-mission-and-values accessed 26 March 2023
[2] Australian International School, https://www.ais.ae/about-us/vision-mission-and-values accessed 26 March 2023

of that, and children from vastly different cultures were expected to communicate with each other as any children anywhere would.

Learning music can be made enjoyable for most children, and they respond readily, making communication with each other fun.

I had not envisaged teaching such a large variety of children. They were from vastly different cultures, and some spoke very little or no English. I could easily have had Russian, Sri Lankan, Indian, Emirati, Australian, and European students in the one class. It was very interesting working in such an environment. I needed to be ever mindful of the different customs and religious beliefs of my multi-cultural students.

I spoke no other languages, so if my English and physical gestures were not understood, I just moved on with the lesson. We muddled along, which sounds a bit flippant, but it feels right to say this because I was learning too—how to teach well, such a wide variety of students.

There were of course a few children who already spoke English. They were undoubtedly a boon to their

Chapter Two:
Leaving Home

classmates and by the end of that first year all my students were speaking functional English.

English was the first language of the teaching staff, so communication with the adults was easy. Regarding staff members though, we were expected to dress conservatively, sleeves (at least t-shirt length), and hems below the knees. I often wore three quarter length sleeves for good measure. Conservative dress was one thing, a bit like going back to the 1960s, a time I hadn't experienced, though I'd seen photos, of course. But coming from North Queensland where *no one* wore much, to *having* to wear clothes that covered most of my skin was strange and challenging. It took me a while to become accustomed to it, particularly in the relentless heat.

Down Time

Something in the UAE that differed vastly from Australia, was the consumption of alcohol. In principle, it was prohibited in the Emirates because of strict adherence to Sharia Law, however regulations varied from one Emirate to the next and authorities often overlooked the use of alcohol where tourists or expats were concerned. It is worth noting, these laws have now relaxed considerably. (Significant changes occurred on 7 November 2020 under a federal law change, and a further change was announced by Dubai lawmakers on 1 January 2023. **Consumption of alcohol is no longer a criminal offense,** and a license fee is no longer required for residents or tourists.[3])

However, in some areas when I lived there, such as Ras Al Khaimah, Ajman, Umm Al Quwain and Fujairah, the purchase and consumption of alcohol was unproblematic providing you were over the age of twenty-one and not a Muslim.

There was a housing development north of us, in Umm al-Quwain. I travelled there occasionally accompanied by others, but never alone. There was a house on this estate which looked like any of its neighbours, but it was different in one respect. It comprised a shop with ample alcohol for sale. We called this house The Hole in The

---

[3] Dubai Travel Planner, *Is it Okay for Me to Drink Alcohol in UAE? 2 Jan, 2023* https://www.dubaitravelplanner.com/drinking-alcohol-in-dubai, Accessed 9 Jun 2023

Chapter Two:
Leaving Home

Wall and on these infrequent, but clandestine visits we always bought enough to last some months.

Had we been caught with alcohol the consequences could have been severe. Whipping as a penalty was still in the UAE criminal code for drunkenness, though I, personally, knew of no one who had endured this awful punishment. Loss of license, a significant fine, or imprisonment for public alcohol consumption were alternate consequences if they were caught.[4]

Arguably, the most shameful punishment for a woman in my position was deportation. Prudently, my friends and I were discreet. We surreptitiously drank, as much as the next person, but in the privacy of our homes. I appreciated the opportunity to be in the UAE and wasn't going to do anything to jeopardise my stay.

---

[4] Strohal, Theodor, Strohal Legal Group, *Can I Get You Another Glass? – Dos and Don'ts Around The Alcohol Consumption in the UAE* https://www.slg-strohallegalgroup.com accessed 18 Apr 2023

Moving On

After a year teaching at AIS Sharjah, I moved to Dubai and worked there for the following two years. I lived alone in an apartment, which the Dubai British School paid for, and once again taught music to enthusiastic students. I taught piano privately as well, to fund further travels later. The British school was more western than the previous Sharjah posting, with primarily British expat kids, though some came from elsewhere in the world, including the surrounding Arabic countries.

Life in Dubai

Life was western in Dubai. Commonwealth citizens were free to roam at will, but I adhered to conservative dress everywhere, including work, even though the school was British. Once again, all the Commonwealth teachers respected the conservative dress code. I was never disrespected by the UAE nationals, in fact, the Emirati men in particular, were very courteous to me.

In this region of the world 'stuff got done' at an astonishing rate. I witnessed a spaghetti flyover, criss-crossing roads, built over Sheikh Zayed Road, within a

Chapter Two:
Leaving Home

week. What a pity red tape and, to a degree, a laissez-faire attitude thwarts this kind of rapid progress in Australia. I couldn't help but notice how hard and fast people worked in the UAE. There is an attitude of 'we want it done, so it will get done'.

I was working hard in my way. Singing for my students was mandatory in my classes and I sang so much that eventually my voice began to feel the strain. I recognised it would be wise to seek help.

There was little need for me to seek medical assistance while in the UAE. In my mid-twenties, and healthy, this wasn't surprising. I also dated a man who was in the medical field. His aunt was one of the world's leading acupuncturists, so I was mingling with quite open-minded people who found relevance in alternative, as well as conventional, medicines.

In my search for someone to help me when I did need it, I encountered EFT Tapping. I tried it and found it useful. In fact, I was so impressed by EFT, I undertook the first-level course in the discipline to ensure I could successfully treat myself. Thankfully, the outcome for my voice was positive. So too was Tapping helpful in my classroom. I employed EFT occasionally, and achieved pleasing results, with nervous performers.

Three years teaching in the UAE, and I had made friends that would stay with me always. The entire experience was so valuable particularly regarding enhancing my appreciation for other cultures and my tolerance for teaching under extraordinary circumstances.

Chapter Three: Settling Down

Going Home

Call it instinct, divine intervention or what you will, but in time, Dubai told me it was time to leave. It's extraordinary how a person *just knows* these things. It may have had something to do with the desire to realise another of my goals – to find a life partner. The men I had dated in the UAE all wanted to remain in the northern hemisphere. I wanted to return home to Australia.

When I left the Arabian Desert, I was outwardly a conservative girl, so coming back to Australia's Gold Coast where everyone dressed in the least that was legal, ensured I had tremendous difficulty readjusting. But I did, eventually, and as I resumed life as an Australian in my homeland, I began to think about the goal I'd come home to achieve. It was time I found a partner to share my life with.

A new way of meeting people had emerged while I'd been busy living my dream. Online dating. Goodness what a challenge. Would I get it right?

I did. I found Richard online, met him in person in 2011, and soon recognised that in this man I would have the ideal mate. He was a warm, lovely natured man with a good heart. I felt I'd picked a sensible man with a positive attitude and a loyal and committed work ethic. I decided that this was the man I'd marry.

A Wedding

My parents were still in our family home, so Richard and I arranged for our wedding to take place between Warwick and my Gold Coast home. My sister/bridesmaid and Dad were with me when I dressed and left from a Mt Tambourine hotel to meet my fiancé. The hairdresser had insisted I sit for hours with rollers in, but some of my friends came around during that time, so thankfully I had some good company.

It was a three o'clock ceremony on December 8^{th,} 2012; a glorious afternoon, in what was then called, The Heritage Estate Winery.

Chapter Three:
Settling Down

The property was home to a splendid building that was once the old church in Burleigh Heads. It had been transported up the mountain and was now run as a wedding venue by good people with excellent experience. Everything was provided except the music. We engaged a harpist for the church because my mother liked the instrument and we hired a jazz band for the entertainment and their performance was fabulous. Warm lighting and twinkling candelabras contributed to the cosy ambiance. There was a stairway that went nowhere; though the recently wed could descend it; their first entrance as the newly married couple. It was gorgeous.

I enjoyed being the princess for the day. Richard and I sat on our own because we couldn't decide who to have on the bridal table. Apparently, we started a trend!

The venue's proprietors decanted on our table, a luscious port, and Richard drank more than was prudent. I could only manage one wine, but I had a smile so wide my face hurt by the end of the day. We had thoroughly enjoyed ourselves.

Two months later, we took a honeymoon in Bali. Neither of us had been there before and though the people were lovely we have never been inspired to repeat the experience.

Kids of Our Own

I had been teaching for sixteen years before I deferred for three years to have our two children. The first, Matthew, was a very unsettled baby. I don't think I knew quite what hit me. I was good with kids, but an unsettled baby was something I'd never encountered. It was difficult and undermined my belief in myself. I was operating on auto pilot.

Two years and three weeks after Matthew was born, Jemma burst into the world a happier, more contented child than her brother. Apart from Matthew's consistent discontent and tantrums to express himself, I enjoyed having babies, but as toddlers, they kept me vigilant.

Jemma, always interested in the world around her, walked at ten months' and simply didn't stop. Matthew remained unsettled with more meltdowns than I could count. I questioned my ability to manage my children. It

Chapter Three:
Settling Down

was more about survival. I was always on edge waiting for the next Matthew meltdown. I felt I had no control or influence over his anxiety, though I'm certain I spoke calmly and clearly to him, despite my frayed nerves. He'd never have understood his world had I not been calm with him.

As he has matured, I have seen him respond positively to different strategies his teachers and I have taught him for dealing with his anxiety. It's such a joy to see him working out how to cope, and it's much better when we are not being reactive to his angry, spontaneous outbursts. It is draining on my energy and mental health, as each outburst must be interpreted and dealt with on its own merit.

I knew meltdowns in children were communication, but Matthew was yet to learn that his way of communicating didn't always convey his intended message. An intervention I'd tried previously on a particular behaviour, didn't necessarily work on subsequent presentations of that same behaviour. I had to continually think of something new to divert him. We simply learned together.

Richard's Ventures

And what of Richard through this challenging period? When Matthew was a baby, Richard was the Managing Director of his family's business, Aviation Ground Handling.

Ground handling companies exist to provide services to the aviation industry. Employees undertake an astonishing number of tasks to facilitate effective handling of people, baggage, and aircraft within an airport. They deal daily with everything from providing a wheelchair for a disabled traveller to repositioning aircraft on the tarmac. Even when the family sold AGH to the Gold Coast Airport, Richard stayed on as General Manager.

In 2013, the Gold Coast Airport sold Aviation Ground Handling to a competitor company. Until then, the business had retained the name Richard's family gave it, but now that significant changes, including a new business name, were afoot, my hard-working husband looked for an alternative career.

Chapter Three:
Settling Down

I was certainly open to something new. We only had Matthew at that stage. I was coping better with him and was open to a change with a challenge. A move out west where we had secured the franchise of the Quest Apartment Hotel in Ipswich was ideal. Purchasing this was within our budget and would take me closer to my sister. I was looking forward to seeing her more often, and having her support as a young mother, as indeed, I could also be to her.

The training Richard and I undertook for this jointly owned apartment management franchise, was insufficient, but my enthusiasm, my husband's competent business skills, his expertise with people and great staff already at the Quest, were a winning combination. Though the experience presented us with a very steep learning curve, we were more than up to the task. Besides, if anyone would make a business a success, Richard would. He's superb.

When we took over the Quest, Matthew was fifteen months old, and just as we began work, we realised we were expecting our second baby. This meant that my new career was short-lived, but Jemma was a wonderful reason to give up work for a while. Richard ran the Quest so capably that I didn't need to worry at all.

We built the business to greater than it was when we bought it, and we sold at a reasonable profit. It transpired it was very lucky we did. COVID-19 happened soon after and there was a probability of failure had we tried to remain in business through this period.

My career had been put on hold when I worked with Richard and while I was establishing a routine with my children. I was exhausted. I simply couldn't have gone back to teaching any sooner than I did. Breastfeeding a baby while working out of the home is rarely ideal. Add that to Matthew's unsettled behaviour, to which we could now add night terrors, leaving him sleep deprived, ensured a less-than-ideal situation for everyone.

Another Move

In late 2019, we moved to Brisbane. We bought a gorgeous house with abundant natural light, in a leafy street, overlooking a park. Brisbane has always had excellent recreational areas, and the expansive park over our back fence was no exception. It boasted an excellent

Chapter Three:
Settling Down

playground, an abandoned mine (therefore an interesting history) and a restful brook which bubbled along at the bottom of the cliff at the end of our yard. Another goal achieved and life was good.

Then I found a lump.

Chapter Four:
Finding a Lump

The Cancer Journey

Where there was no lump the day before, there was one now and it grew two inches overnight. I'm a tall, slender lady with small breasts, so I could not miss this lump.

I hoped it was a cyst. I simply did not know what could grow as rapidly as this mass did.

But I knew it was a problem.

It was utterly astonishing how quickly it appeared, how large it grew, and though I wasn't to know it yet, how profoundly it would change my life.

I wasn't an ardently religious person, but I prayed about this lump. The whole idea of breast cancer when I was so young and the mother of two small children was confronting and overwhelming. Yes, of course, I knew seeing a specialist was a certainty, but I needed some time to process what might be happening; time to investigate other options before the inevitable whirlwind of conventional medical treatment. I spent the best part of a fortnight cogitating over what those different options might be.

Alternative Therapies

I had always been open to alternative ideas regarding healing. It might have been God's intervention, (or at least some force bigger than me) that led me to discover German New Medicine.

German New Medicine came to my attention while browsing the net. Pioneered by Dr Ryka Geerd Hamer, he maintained GNM 'was *not only a new paradigm of medicine but also a new consciousness. It is the awareness that our organism* (our body) *possesses inexhaustible creativity and remarkable self-healing capabilities. It is the recognition that each cell of our body is endowed with a biological wisdom we share with all living beings.*[5]

---

[5] Hamer, Ryka G., Markolin,C., *German New Medicine*, www.learningGNM.com accessed 16 March, 2023

Chapter Four:
Finding a Lump

Yes, I believed in the body's capacity to self-heal when the conditions were at their most favourable.

Non-invasive therapies, those that promoted the body's capacity to heal itself, were always going to pique my interest, and I was more than ready to explore what was available for serious physical maladies. I was certain there was more I could do for myself than simply rely on the painful and invasive conventional methods of dealing with what could quite possibly be cancer. Perhaps some might think me irresponsible for not screaming out for an immediate appointment with an oncologist. But so immensely confronting was this potentially serious illness over which I appeared to have no control, I had to give myself time to digest it first. I needed to consider what the best course of action *for me* would be.

Pursuing Something Different

It was August 2021. I had been following a global Facebook page which promoted community bonding of the group participants, both with each other, and with like-minded people in their own locality—wherever in the world they lived. The administration would sometimes conduct meditations for the page participants. People often found clarity or direction through talking with other group members or participating in the meditations.

Belonging to this group had nothing to do with my health. I'd been a member for some time before the lump appeared. I simply liked the aspirations, attitudes, and anecdotes I was hearing from the participants.

Drawn to innovations, I attended a fortnightly meeting with the closest group participants in proximity to me. If its members were enjoying this global Facebook page and listening to the same uplifting podcasts as I was, I wanted to meet them.

Lisa Brough

Lisa Brough and her partner were hosting the meetup in their home. Lisa had considerable knowledge and experience with alternative therapies, and she knew much more about cancer than I did. I was buoyed by our interaction. She was familiar with Dr Hamer's work and talking with her about GNM led to a discussion on Biomagnetism.

Chapter Four:
Finding a Lump

Prior to that day, I hadn't heard of Biomagnetism. However, the more I listened to Lisa, the more I realised, as a practitioner of this treatment, she was offering the answer to my prayer. By the time I left her home I had decided to book appointments for her to treat me.

Chapter Five:
Finding Biomagnetism

The Beginning of my Journey with Biomagnetism

Choosing to try Biomagnetism wasn't a giant leap into the unknown for me. I had tried multiple alternative therapies, with varying degrees of success. Over the years, I'd used acupuncture, kinesiology, chiropractic, energy healing in a variety of formats, including reiki, intuitive massage, homeopathy, flower essences, hypnotherapy and other combined approaches. I had once trained in Level 1 EFT, *which focuses on tapping the 12 meridian points of the body to relieve symptoms of a negative experience or emotion.*[6] I'd also had a short-lived but effective session of EMDR therapy[i] so I knew my body

---

[6] Anthony, K., Healthline, *EFT Tapping*, https://www.healthline.com/health/eft-tapping accessed 16 March, 2023

iEMDR Therapy involves 'eye movement desensitization and reprocessing. It is a psychotherapy treatment technique developed by Dr Francine Shapiro PhD designed to ease the distress associated with traumatic memories responded well to some alternative therapies. I was in no doubt I wanted to give Biomagnetism a go.

What is Biomagnetism?

Biomagnetism is a non-invasive therapeutic technique based on the dysfunction of two specific anatomical points.[7]

It is a therapy for the prevention, diagnosis, and treatment of diseases using static magnetic fields.[8]

Biomagnetism therapy uses pairs of medium intensity static magnets to balance the body's pH levels to allow healing. The Biomagnetic Pair is created by an imbalance in the alkalinity or acidity of the tissue that supports it. This imbalance has created a pathology or dysfunction. The Biomagnetic Pair always has a vibrational and energetic resonance.

---

[7]de Castro Cossenza, C.A., et la, Saude Coletiva, Revista FT, Volume 27 *Medicinal Biomgnetism – Level 1 and Level 2 Biomagnetic Pairs Scanning Methodology, https://revistaft.com.br/, 2023*
[8]Viapiana, C., et al, Research Gate, *Fundamentals of Medicinal Biomagentism,* March 2023 *https://www.researchgate.net/publication/369044123_FUNDAMENTALS_OF_MEDICINAL_BIOMAGNETISM* accessed 25 July 2024

Chapter Five:
Finding Biomagnetism

To further distinguish Biomagnetism, it is often referred to as Biomagnetic Pair Therapy (BMP).

My First Biomagnetism Appointments

I instinctively liked and trusted Lisa Brough. At the first appointment, I climbed onto her table with hope; I had no reservations at all. I was confident Biomagnetism was a way forward, and this was the woman who would help me proceed.

Whilst still working and managing the family, I prioritised five appointments with Lisa over a six-week period. With each successive session, the progress gave me the impetus to continue.

After this course of treatment, I found the lump had diminished to **half** its original size.

That was astonishing.

I wanted to understand how this occurred, and as I became better informed, I was determined to train in the discipline.

This therapy was life-changing for me, and I wanted to tell the world.

Conventional Medicine

Most people avail themselves of conventional medicine because it's what they've always known. Many don't realise it treats the symptoms, not the cause. Often though, once they've tried an alternative therapy, and experienced advancement, or success, they're more likely to continue with it and more open to trying others if the need arises.

I'd had a marvellous experience with Biomagnetism. However, I knew my loved ones would be expecting me to investigate conventional treatments as well. Reluctantly, I sought a referral and booked into an oncologist.

The Conventional Medicine Journey

I struggled with every step of the conventional medicine process. It was all so confronting. In the late afternoon before my surgery, after I'd had some nuclear dye

Chapter Five:
Finding Biomagnetism

injected into my nipple, I met my breast care nurse and cried.

Copiously.

I just wasn't sure that all that was happening to me was *really* necessary. The dye had been injected with a very fine needle. It was uncomfortable but not excruciating. This procedure highlighted where my sentinel lymph nodes were, so the surgeon knew which nodes to remove.

My first surgery to remove my breast revealed a 2.5cm cancerous tumour, along with more than 35 satellite tumours throughout the breast tissue. It would be a long wait to see if there was cancer in the sentinel lymph nodes, too. If there was, it would mean a second surgery to remove all lymph nodes and further discussions on my future treatment plan.

The pathology results were devastating. There was cancer in the lymph nodes. I cried again. Even more than previously. I was crying with extreme sadness that the cancer had spread beyond what had been removed. And I cried because I had more treatment to endure, in whatever way that manifested. Thankfully, my best friend was with me to comfort me when I received this news.

Two weeks later, I underwent lymph node clearance surgery, followed by the recommended chemotherapy and radiation therapy. I seriously struggled with the chemo and radiation, partly because they were horrendous to endure physically, and partly because they were emotionally draining. Radiation therapy was the most challenging. The fatigue was mind and body numbing, especially when I still had to be a wife and a mother, with limited immediate support to my four- and six-year-old children. Now, I was feeling hideous, and absolutely everything about my life was uncertain.

But I persisted until the treatment was completed.

I had even changed my diet to ensure I wasn't ingesting toxins that could promote ill health—or that my body didn't need. And I was working through any possible emotional issues that may have triggered the dis-ease as well.

I know the surgery removed all the cancer, but to this day, I'm not convinced the chemo, and particularly the

Chapter Five:
Finding Biomagnetism

radiation therapy killed any cancer. Not for me personally. I truly don't believe there was any left to kill, but since cancer is so awful, I did see the sense in attacking it with multiple disciplines and I knew it put my family's minds at ease that I pursued the conventional road. It's simply that chemo and radiation are so toxic, and I very clearly didn't need or want to feel so miserable when I led such a busy life.

My last radiation treatment was on my 44th birthday.

Regeneration

Within six weeks after the last treatment, my hair began to grow back. In fact, I had a cute new hairdo because it emerged in curly swathes. However, it was months before I began to feel physically and psychologically regenerated. Though I was minus a breast, (and that was something else to deal with), eventually I began to feel relief in the healing process.

Leaving chemo and radiation behind meant I could now resume the Biomagnetism I had previously found so beneficial. Not only did I want to continue with this therapy, but I had become passionate about it and was eager to train as a therapist to bring it to others as well.

I began another learning journey.

PART II

MAGNETS AND HEALING

What Modalities Paved the Way for the Discovery of the Biomagnetism I'd Become Passionate About?

Knowing the answer to this question would help me to understand why and how Biomagnetism developed. But before looking at the research that directly influenced the discovery of Biomagnetism, let's consider briefly, the history of magnet therapies.

A Short History of Magnet Modalities

Magnet therapies date back thousands of years. *The Yellow Emperor's Book of Internal Medicine*, recorded around 2000 BC and considered to be the world's earliest medical textbook, describes the application of lodestone, the earth's only natural magnet, to the body's energy channels, or meridians, to treat unbalances.[9]

---

[9] Anderson E. Z., Caro-Scarpitto, C., Science Direct, *Complementary Therapies for Physical Therapy, Magnets*, 2008, https://www.sciencedirect.com/topics/medicine-and-dentistry/magnet-therapy accessed 26 May 2023

Vedas, the religious scriptures of the Hindus, is another ancient text that includes descriptions of using devices thought to have been made of lodestone.[10]

The writings of the ancient Greeks and Egyptians gave evidence of their belief in the healing properties of magnets and their use of them in treating a variety of disorders.

Through the centuries, physicians continued to employ magnets in their treatments. The Swiss physician Paracelsus (1493-1541) believed the mind and body were interconnected through a life force (which he called 'archaeus'). He proposed archaeus was influenced by the forces found in magnets. Magnets could therefore be used to treat illness and promote self-healing.[11]

---

[10] Anderson E. Z., Caro-Scarpitto, C., Science Direct, *Complementary Therapies for Physical Therapy, Magnets*, 2008, https://www.sciencedirect.com/topics/medicine-and-dentistry/magnet-therapy accessed 26 May 2023

[11] Anderson E. Z., Caro-Scarpitto, C., Science Direct, *Complementary Therapies for Physical Therapy, Magnets*, 2008, https://www.sciencedirect.com/topics/medicine-and-dentistry/magnet-therapy accessed 26 May 2023

Magnets and Healing

During the next century, William Gilbert, physician to Queen Elizabeth I, perpetuated the use of magnets to promote health and treat illness.

By the middle of the eighteenth century, the public's interest in the healing properties of magnets had grown. Maximilian Hell, a Hungarian-born Jesuit priest and astronomer achieved good results with his clients. Hell's ideas significantly influenced Anton Mesmer, a physician and scientist who was trained in medicine, mathematics, and law.[12]

Mesmer believed in a universal life force and coined the term 'animal magnetism' to describe the force in living creatures. However, although Mesmer was popular with the public and treated many people, his belief regarding the use of the energy concentrated in magnets, defined as mineral magnetism, coupled with his own animal magnetism, to cure clients' ailments prompted strong criticism from medical authorities.[13]

---

[12] Anderson E. Z., Caro-Scarpitto, C., Science Direct, *Complementary Therapies for Physical Therapy, Magnets*, 2008, https://www.sciencedirect.com/topics/medicine-and-dentistry/magnet-therapy accessed 26 May 2023

[13] ibid

As Mesmer's popularity in Europe waned, interest in magnet therapy grew in the United States. Here proponents of magnet therapy and makers of magnetic products including hats, belts and insoles continued into the early twentieth century with little support from the established medical community. Magnetic blankets were also popular. People reported benefits such as perceived increased blood flow and a reduction in pain and inflammation in areas of dis-ease when using these items.

Advances in surgical procedures and successes using antibiotic therapy eventually saw magnet therapy move into the shadows.[14]

The Research That Directly Influenced the Discovery of Biomagnetism

Dr Linus Pauling

In the 1930s, American Dr Linus Pauling, researching in both theoretical and applied medicine, made important discoveries in an astonishing number of disciplines, but

---

[14] Anderson E. Z., Caro-Scarpitto, C., Science Direct, *Complementary Therapies for Physical Therapy, Magnets*, 2008, https://www.sciencedirect.com/topics/medicine-and-dentistry/magnet-therapy accessed 26 May 2023

most particularly in chemistry—physical, structural, analytical, inorganic, and organic chemistry, and in biochemistry. A little later, he became interested in the highly complex molecules within living organisms.

He was a deserving recipient of the 1954 Nobel Prize for Chemistry for discovering the **magnetic properties in blood.**[15]

Albert Roy Davis and Walter Rawls

In 1991 Dr Richard Broeringmeyer noted that in 1936, Albert Roy Davis and Walter Rawls, had demonstrated the effects of the north and south poles of magnets on blood, nerve, bacteria and plant cells.

Davis and Rawls had showed that cells' biological activity increased with a magnetic field application. Thus arose the approximation between biology and magnetism.[16]

---

[15] Oregon State University, Linus Pauling Institute, *Linus Pauling Biography*, 2023 https://lip.oregonstate.edu/about/linuspauling-biography accessed 05 August 2023

[16] de Castro Cossenza, C.A., et la, Saude Coletiva, Revista FT, Volume 27 *Medicinal Biomgnetism – Level 1 and Level 2 Biomagnetic Pairs Scanning Methodology*, https://revistaft.com.br/, 2023 accessed 5 August 2023

Dr Kyoichi Nakagawa

Dr Kyoichi Nakagawa published an influential study in which he described the human body as being 'essentially a large electromagnetic field that operates under the influence of electrically charged ions'.

He talked about the nervous system being, **'in part, controlled by changing patterns of ions and electromagnetic fields.** Every thought or action, therefore, caused the electric transfer of signals from the brain to the corresponding limb'.

The existence of every cell in the human body is based on electricity. **'A disturbance of the magnetic balance brings about dysfunction of the cells, causing diseases, pain, mental or emotional problems, insomnia and other bodily imbalances,'** he wrote.

Dr Nakagawa determined that the decline of earth's magnetic field caused people to suffer symptoms such as fatigue, insomnia, dizziness and other generalised aches and pains. Naming the condition Magnetic Field Deficiency Syndrome (MFDS), he found that the external application of a magnetic field to the human body would ease the symptoms of MFDS. Western medicine's version of chronic fatigue syndrome and fibromyalgia seem to correlate very closely with MFDS.[17]

Dr Richard Broeringmeyer

In the 1980s, Dr Richard Broeringmeyer was the medical director at NASA. Noticing all astronauts returned to the earth with one leg shorter than the other, he sought to investigate organic dysfunctions in bodies of space explorers.

He achieved the measurement of Biomagnetic Poles generated by abnormal concentration of hydrogen ions that, outside their normal values (magnetic polarisation), cause dysfunctions in affected organs.

He also studied the effects the lack of gravity had on astronauts. This led him to experiment by balancing their bodies with magnets. He suggested a cause for the

---

[17]PMEF Therapy Australia, Understanding Magnetic Field Deficiency Syndrome (MFDS) https://pemf.com.au/magnetic-field-deficiency-syndrome/ accessed 11 August 2023

anomaly of short leg syndrome could be the lack of Earth's magnetic field in space.[18]

It is also well documented that a healthy cell in the body rotates to the left while its nucleus rotates to the right, thus creating energy. The diseased cell rotates to the right and its nucleus turns to the left. While the healthy cell produces energy, the diseased or unhealthy cell takes energy away from the body to give to the disease. In theory, as the disease worsens, more and more energy is required from the body's reserves to survive. When most of the body's reserves are depleted by disease, death is imminent. Reversing the turn of the diseased cell conserves energy drainage and helps the body fight the disease.[19]

Since magnets could alter the electric potential within biological tissue, the conclusion presented itself that magnets could re-implement a disrupted balance of bio-

---

[18] Broeringmeyer, Dr. R., Biomagnetic Pair Therapy, *Principles of Magnetic Therapy*, https://biomagnetismesdona.com/dr-richard-broeringmeyer/ accessed 29 June 2024

[19] Broeringmeyer, Dr. R. Principios De La Terapia Magnetica, *Biomagnetismo*, Self Published by Dr. Richard Broeringmeyer and Dr Mary Droeringmeyer, 1978

electric potential, one which created a foundation for the development of pathological states.[20]

In 1988, in a course promoted by the Guadalajara Society of Alternative Medicines Dr Broeringmeyer laid out the foundations of what he called Energy Therapy, in which the Static Magnetic Fields combined with kinesiology could scan the body using an electromagnet.[21]

In attendance at this course was Mexican surgeon Dr Isaac Goiz Duran.

Dr Isaac Goiz Duran (The Father of Biomagnetism and a man to whom the world owes so much.)

It was at this course that surgeon, acupuncturist and physiotherapist, Dr Issac Goiz Duran was inspired by Dr Broeringmeyer's research to conduct further investigation into the impact of single pole magnetic

---

[20] Broeringmeyer, Dr. R., Biomagnetic Pair Therapy, *Principles of Magnetic Therapy,* https://biomagnetismesdona.com/dr-richard-broeringmeyer/ accessed 29 June 2024
[21] Nazareth Franco, A. L. et al, RevistaFT, Ciencias da Saude, Volume 27, *The Use of Medicinal Biomagnetism for Chronic Venous Insufficiency-Lower Limbs Blood Flow Protocol,* https://revistaft.com. accessed 15 July 2024

fields on living organisms. He also determined to find that which he believed *must* exist: **Biomagnetic Pairs**.[22] This intuitive belief would prove profound.

What is a Biomagnetic Pair?

Biomagnetic Pairs (BMP) comprise the bi-focal relation between two disease-causing points of the body. BMPs are created when there are two specific areas in the body that are energetically connected and resonating with each other. One is positive-acidic, the other negative-alkaline.[23]

These imbalances cause dysfunctions and symptoms affecting the body. The health of unbalanced areas is restored by balancing the acid and alkaline levels of the body when applying medium intensity magnets of opposite polarity to those specific areas.[24]

---

[22] Pilarinos, D., Biomagnetic Health, *Dr Isaac Goiz Duran and the History of Biomagnetism* 27 September 2021, https://www.biomaghealth.com/post/dr-goiz-biomagnetism-magnets accessed 24 June 2024

[23] Guerrero, H., Biomagnetism USA, *What is a Biomagnetic Pair?* http://www.biomagnetismusa.com/ accessed 15 March 2023

[24] Ibid

Every illness is caused by either internal or external toxicity from different sources. **This toxicity causes a pH imbalance of tissue and internal organs.**[25]

Since Dr Goiz discovered the first Biomagnetic Pair (the thymus and the rectum, in 1988) and developed the therapy to treat his patients, he and other clinicians have researched and discovered hundreds of Biomagnetic pairs.[26]

The Advantages of Biomagnetism

One of the significant advantages of Biomagnetism is that, like Magnetic Resonance Imaging, (which was also pioneered in the 1980s) it is non-invasive. Whereas MRI is used to map the internal structure and certain aspects of function within the body, Biomagnetism can identify and help restore and maintain physical and mental health.

---

[25] Global Biomagnetism, Todos Los Derechos Reservados, What is Biomagnetism? https://globalbiomagnetism.com/about-biomagnetism accessed 14 June 2024

[26] Guerrero, H., Biomagnetism USA, *What is a Biomagnetic Pair?* http://www.biomagnetismusa.com/ accessed 15 March 2023

Bio-magnetism can be combined with other treatments, for example allopathic, which is conventional or western medicine, where the illness is treated with drugs or surgery. It may also be applied with alternative disciplines. **However, Dr Goiz recommended it not be employed for treating a patient who is using intravenous chemotherapy or radiation therapy.** Magnets can also potentially interfere with the efficacy of a pacemaker or internal defibrillator.

The first people Dr Goiz treated were extremely sick AIDS patients. The therapy was so successful that many of those patients outlived the doctor who'd saved them.[27]

Dr Goiz (who died in 2021) trained many clinicians in his discipline including his three sons, Isaac, David and Moises Goiz Martinez. Dr Issac Goiz Duran's Escuela Superior de Biomagnetismo Médico and its highly-trained teachers, as well as Dr Luis Garcia, Helena Guerrero, and Australia's own Lisa Brough, among

---

[27] Unpublished notes from Rosemary Walters to author, accessed 25 July 2024

others throughout the world, continue to provide training in Biomagnetism.

Helena Guerrero CBM, CHT, CMT Holistic Health Specialist

Though Helena Guerrero was one of several clinicians who translated Dr Goiz's work from Spanish to English, it was she who organised for Dr Goiz to provide training in English in the USA in 2010.[28]

Over the next several years, students from Canada, Australia, New Zealand, Ireland and several European countries travelled to the USA to take part in these trainings.

Ms Guerrero's own extensive research has revealed several new Biomagnetic Pairs, two of which were officially recognised by Dr. Goiz. The first pair related to Bartonella bacteria in 2011 and the second came from the discovery of symptoms related to COVID-19 in February 2020.

---

[28] Global Biomagnetism, *Helena Guerrero and Biomagnetism* https://globalbiomagnetism.com/about-us accessed 24 June 2024

Thanks to the increasing availability of online training courses and general worldwide expansion of the therapy, there are now Biomagnetism therapists practicing in more than 20 countries throughout the world.[29]

Is Biomagnetism Like Magnetic Therapy?

Biomagnetism is different from magnetic therapy. The only similarity is the use of magnets. Magnet therapy has been applied with one polar principle just for dysfunction or injuries under two concepts.

a. South pole as analgesic.
b. North pole as anti-inflammatory.

The magnetic fields used are of low intensity between 300 to 5000 gauss and are applied for hours or days.[30]

---

[29] Brough, L., Conference Proceedings and Resources – The Second Annual Australian Biomagnetism Conference, Brough, Lisa, November 19th, 2023 – Biomagnetism Alumni Survey 2023, accessed 26 February 2025

[30] Brough, L., Unpublished notes given to author, accessed 24 July 2024

Magnets and Healing

Examples of this therapy include items such as magnetic blankets, belts for back support and bracelets, as well as static magnets placed on points of discomfort.

There are many configurations of permanent magnets that are commercially available which are used for symptomatic relief.

So far, the placing of singular biomagnetic poles to given areas whose energy is depleted, has resulted in pain relief in up to 70% of applications. Most scientists are aware that magnets have been used for centuries with limited degrees of success. The situation can be corrected now that doctors are aware that the identification of the area to be treated and its biochemistry will define the type of field to be applied.[31]

Why Do Magnets Work?

The human body naturally has magnetic and electric fields. All molecules have a small amount of magnetic energy in them. Illness happens because the body's magnetic fields are out of balance. If the two correct

---

[31] Broeringmeyer, Dr. R. Principios De La Terapia Magnetica, *Biomagnetismo*, Self Published by Dr. Richard Broeringmeyer and Dr Mary Droeringmeyer, 1978

external magnetic fields are put on the body, an imbalance will resolve, and the affected area can return to health.[32]

Davis and Rawls showed that the biological activity of cells increased with the application of a magnetic field. The metallic elements and ions in the cell, when exposed to a north pole, decreased the biological effects and reduced its activity. When applied to unhealthy cells, it produced a relaxed condition similar to the body's defence mechanism. When exposed to the south pole, their effects were opposite.[33]

Dr Goiz discovered that medium intensity Biomagnetic fields produced by natural magnets of 1,000 to 15,000 power of attraction (Gauss), **applied in pairs to specific parts of the body that resonate together can balance**

---

[32] Reiff Ellis, R., WebMD, *What is Magnetic Field Therapy?* WebMd LLC 2021 https://www.webmd.com/pain-management/magnetic-field-therapy-overview accessed 27 May 2023

[33] de Lacerda Mendes, Dr O., Marcello Gigliotti, Dr J., Editors, Revista FT, Volume 27, *Medicinal Biomgnetism Level 1 and Level 2 Biomagnetic Pairs Scanning Methodology,* 2023 https://revistaft.com.br/medicinal-biomagnetism-level-1-and-level-2-biomagnetic-pairs-scanning-methodology/ accessed 14 July 2024

the pH of an unbalanced area. This allows for the body to restore itself to health.

In 33 years of practice, Dr Goiz identified 350 Biomagnetic Pairs that cover most of the glandular dysfunctions, diseases, syndromes and illnesses such as diabetes, cancer, HIV and Covid. He found that common diseases were produced by a single Biomagnetic Pair (BMP) and complex diseases were the result of the presence of two or more BMPs.[34]

Dr Goiz treated more than 500,000 patients with Biomagnetism and trained more than 20,000 Medical Doctors and other Health Therapists from many countries. In 1999, he was awarded a PhD in Bio-energetic Medicine from England's Oxford International University.[35]

The Identification of the Biomagnetic Pairs in Each Patient

---

[34] Guerrero, H., Biomagnetism USA, http://www.biomagnetismusa.com/ accessed 20 June 2024
[35] Bossa, C. V., et al, Editora Academica Periodicojs Health and Society, Vol 3 *Fundamentals of Medicinal Biomagnetism,* 2023 https://www.researchgate.net/accessed 21 Jun 2024

Identification occurs through a physical screening known as a Biomagnetic and Bioenergetic scan.

When an area of imbalance in acidity or alkalinity is present, the right side of the body contracts, which is observed most clearly in the feet, the legs being the longest leavers of the body, therefore showing the most differentiation.

The client relaxes on the massage table and the practitioner places a negative magnet on a specific area of the body, states its biomagnetic reference name (e.g. liver or wrist etc), and lifts the legs slightly upward, looking for the right side shortening. If the leg shortens on a particular point, the therapist places the negative magnet on that point and then places a positive magnet on the corresponding resonating point, which neutralises the BMP, evening out the legs. The therapist then continues to scan the body for the next BMP.

The biomagnetism therapist is also able to detect where emotional imbalances have impacted on the physical well-being of the client, and specific placement of the magnets can provide improvements in these areas.

Magnets and Healing

Magnets are placed throughout the treatment and left on the body for the required time. At the end of the treatment the client feels relaxed and fabulous and is better able to continue with their day. Over subsequent hours and days the client notices improvements in their health condition.[36]

Magnets Alone Do Not Heal.

It needs to be understood that magnets themselves do not heal. When speaking of Biomagnetism, only when placed in opposing polarities in pairs on specific areas of the body do magnets establish the conditions for the body to heal itself.

pH imbalances are highlighted when the vibrational energy created by the magnets screening the body identifies them. The imbalances cause dysfunctions and symptoms affecting the body.[37]

---

[36] Walters, R.J., Unpublished notes given to the author, 24 July 2024, accessed 25 July 2024
[37] Global Biomagnetism Todos Los Derechos Reservados, 2021, *What is Biomagnetism?* https://globalbiomagnetism.com/about-biomagnetism

The Magnets

The magnets used in Biomagnetism are of medium intensity at a minimum of 1,000 gauss to heal, and the time of application for optimum results varies from ten to thirty minutes. (It is worth noting here, that if a person is treated in the thirteen countries through which the equator passes, their results occur more quickly. The further away from the equator, the longer the therapy takes to work.)

The Biggest Formal Study That Demonstrates the Efficacy of Biomagnetism

In May 2009, Dr. Raymond Hilu, a leading world-renowned cellular biologist[38] invited Dr Goiz to conduct with him a 'before and after' study of 256 patients at Dr. Hilu's clinic in Malaga, Spain.

Dr Hilu MD and his colleague, Dr. Santiago de la Rosa MD, were as objective as possible by inviting patients from various countries. Participants came from USA, England, Germany, France, Sweden, Finland, India and

---

[38]Dr Raymond Hilu, 2020 https://thehiluinstitute.com/about/, accessed 25 July 2023

Spain. There were also many medical doctors invited to observe. Among those present were Dr. Conte MD, and Dr. Limonti MD, from Italy and Dr. Mary Staggs MD from England.[39] All patients suffered from very serious health conditions.

A blood sample was taken from the patients prior to being diagnosed and treated by Dr Goiz with the Biomagnetic Pairs. Another sample was taken after the therapy, to check if the microorganisms indicated as present in their pathologies were still present in the blood after treatment. The results were outstanding.[40] The study's findings were an especially powerful example of Biomagnetism's impact on the blood and its ability to mitigate Rouleaux formations (when red blood cells "stick together" to form chains and stacks) with the placement of just a few magnetic pairs.[41]

---

[39] Global Biomagnetism, *Biomagnetic Pair Tested at Clinic in Spain*, https://globalbiomagnetism.com/clinical-studies accessed 25 July 2024

[40] Global Biomagnetism, *Biomagnetic Pair Tested at Clinic in Spain*, https://globalbiomagnetism.com/clinical-studies accessed 25 July 2024

[41] Pilarinos, D., Biomagnetic Health, *Dr Isaac Goiz Duran and the History of Biomagnetism*, 27 Sept. 2021,

Dr Hilu reported that the study *'was an absolute success. Biomagnetism is one of the most efficient therapies I've encountered in all the years I've practiced Medicine. The most surprising aspect is its simplicity. And an immense advantage, is that it has no side effects.'* [42]

A Second Study

Dr Bryan L. Franke established a pilot study which *'examined the laboratory responses of patients with laboratory-documented typhoid fever who were treated with Biomagnetic Pair Therapy (BPT; medical biomagnetism), a specific application of pairs of magnets for various ailments that are infectious and otherwise.'*

Materials and Methods: The study was an assessment of patients' responses to treatment with only BPT for Salmonella Typhi infections (typhoid fever) using standard conventional laboratory techniques. The research was conducted in an outpatient village clinic in Kenya. There were fifty-two

---

https://www.biomaghealth.com/post/dr-goiz-biomagnetism-magnets acccssed 25 July 2023
[42]Global Biomagnetism, *Biomagnetic Pair Tested at Clinic in Spain* https://globalbiomagnetism.com/clinical-studies accessed 25 July 2024

participants who were evaluated for the possibility of systemic illness, including typhoid fever, from an open-label study. Participants who felt sick and requested testing for possible typhoid fever were tested with a standard Widal test by a certified laboratory technician. Participants who tested positive (13 patients) were then treated with BPT (a 'First Aid' approach) only. These participants then returned for follow-up laboratory and clinical evaluations after 2 days.

Results: Most of the participants (10 of 13) retested as negative, and all patients reported symptomatic clinical improvement.

Conclusions: As a significant majority of participants showed clearing of Salmonella Typhi after BPT, this technique should be studied further in larger trials for its efficacy in treating typhoid fever. [43]

---

[43] Frank, Bryan L., *Biomagnetic Pair Therapy and Typhoid Fever: A Pilot Study,* Medical Acupuncture, 2017 29.5, 308-312, https://www.liebertpub.com/doi/abs/10.1089/acu.2017.1253 accessed 24 July 2023

PART III

STORIES OF SUCCESS

Praise for Rosemary Walters and for Biomagnetism Healing

Rosemary Walters is a warm, engaging human with a passion for helping others. She's practical, no-nonsense, gets things done, and does them well.

As a therapist, the needs of her patient are uppermost in her mind throughout a session, and she doesn't deviate from those needs for a moment.

She will bring restorative healing to anyone who engages her, and she will do so with a charming disposition. Clients will be fortunate indeed to be helped by Rosemary.

~ Rhonda Valentine Dixon

I met Rosemary some years ago and was drawn into her enthusiasm and passion for biomagnetism, spurred on by her own healing journey. I was keen to experience it and noticed several changes within me each time.

1. I always slept very deeply for several days afterward and felt more energised.

2. My elimination was always positively impacted, becoming easier and cleaner.

3. I felt more connected to my body and mind, more grounded.

4. My digestive system was more comfortable.

5. Because Rosemary is asking my body what it needs, different things arise each treatment and it is fascinating to be a witness to what comes up for healing.

6. It is relaxing, calming and restorative on all levels.

I highly recommend Rosemary for her professional approach and her knowledge. She is motivated to make a difference, and her conviction and intent give a potency to her healing ability.

~ Marlene Rutherford

My son Daniel, 9 years old, suffers occasionally from a cold, like any other kid. However, when he became unwell enough to stay home from school, he would invariably get an ear infection and require antibiotics. I was wary of the impact antibiotics

Praise for Rosemary Walters and for Biomagnetism Healing

would have long term, so I decided to get Daniel two biomagnetism treatments each time he became quite unwell with a cold (not just a sniffle). This has happened twice in the last year and Daniel did not get an ear infection either time. Further to this, the second time he seemed to recover much more quickly than previous colds. I am very happy with these results, especially avoiding antibiotics.

~ Rose

Susan's Story

In recent times, I have been through some seriously life-changing events. Throughout the years I've had exposure to several alternative/complimentary therapies, and more recently I was introduced to the concept of Biomagnetism by Rosemary. After hearing of her personal experience, I felt like it was something I wanted to try for myself.

For my initial treatments, my focus was on a calming of my mind and a grounding in my body and a trust that my body would tell Rosemary what it needed. And it did! I left every treatment relaxed and grounded with a good explanation and understanding of what had come up and been treated.

It was a few treatments in when I noticed changes in my digestive system and so that became a focus, as I had planned an overseas trip and didn't want my compromised digestive system to be affected by unfamiliar foods. Again, the treatments provided relief of my symptoms and meant that I was able to fully enjoy my overseas trip.

Susan's Story

Fast forward to returning home, and my symptoms were back and were impacting me greatly. It was around this time that I was diagnosed with Bowel Cancer. Rosemary kept up with regularly treating me and I found this invaluable, both physically and mentally with everything I had going on. I was in such good shape that my surgery went better than the surgeons expected and my recovery from surgery was smooth. I even avoided Influenza A, when four out of the six in my hospital room succumbed!

Unfortunately, it's not the end of my journey with Bowel Cancer just yet, but I am confident that Biomagnetism will continue to help me with my healing journey. I highly recommend Rosemary and the amazing work she does!

Rhonda's Story

For me, years of stress contributed to significant fatigue. I was also tired of trying to optimise my health through diet.

I could manage the stress, but the digestive issues were more difficult.

Eliminating gluten and dairy, lessening my intake of nightshades, reducing my consumption of foods that would compromise my already dodgy immune system AND intermittent fasting all helped. But GPs didn't have the answers. There had to be something that would help me feel healthier and more alive.

When I heard about biomagnetism, I had to try it.

I found the process easy and relaxing, and Rosemary's manner was kind and encouraging. I went away from my first session feeling revitalised. When I was asked how I felt, the words that came to me were, 'the incredible lightness of being'. Unlike the 1984 novel of a similar name which dealt with life being devoid of meaning and the burden of moral or existential weight, my feeling that day was of being unburdened by blocked neural pathways and physical heaviness.

I've had several subsequent beneficial sessions, including one that was a distance healing.

I was busy working one day recently but again fatigued, so I asked Rosemary if she would do a distance healing on me, concentrating on the cortisol level in my body.

I stopped my work, sat down to have lunch and despite not feeling sleepy, not thinking about sleeping and not being aware I might fall asleep, I fell asleep! It was at this time that Rosemary was doing the healing on me. I ALWAYS fall asleep in the physical sessions. I cannot explain falling asleep in the distance session too. It simply happened. Once again, I experienced the 'incredible lightness of being'.

And from there, after the healing, the body can begin to heal itself.

I believe every human would benefit from this extraordinary therapy. Balancing the pH of one's body is common sense, surely.

Lisa Pearson's Story

This is my story of how I came to Biomagnetism.

When my son was 2 years old, he was diagnosed with nephrotic syndrome. No known cause and no known cure only a management plan and cross your fingers he grows out of it by adolescence.

He started off with steroids and then when he became steroid dependant, the next step was to try a stronger medication and the stronger the medication the more his health declined and the more steroids and other medication he needed which ended in a revolving spiral of declining health.

I was not prepared to settle for just managing the condition with allopathic medications, so I began with Chinese herbal medicine. You can imagine how trying to get a 2-year-old to swallow something strong and unpleasant tasting. Needless to say, that was short-lived.

I next went to a naturopath and although these remedies reduced the need for steroids, my son had nine different remedies to take, and some were three times a day or one hour before food and a child eats all the time. And what about when he was at school? I found this to be challenging to keep up with.

I also tried acupuncture, which again maintained better health, however needles were not my son's favourite intervention. It wasn't until my son was sixteen that we found biomagnetism and I wished I had found it sooner. It would have saved him from the trauma of hospital stays, lumbar punctures, rashes, ulcers, papilledema and bullying from other children because of the weight gain from all the medications. There was also the emotional and psychological effect it had on my son and other family members.

What I love about biomagnetism, is that it's just so simple. There are no remedies to take, there is no ridged routine to follow, it's not painful, it is quite relaxing. It didn't contradict any of the medications my son was taking. It is a simple treatment that can easily be maintained for chronic conditions after initial treatments.

Lisa Brough's Story

I became aware of Biomagnetism as part of my own healing journey in 2013. After having my beautiful family – 3 children in 5 years, I developed all the symptoms of a low functioning thyroid. Low body temperature, extreme weight gain of 26kg in a short period of time and crushing fatigue despite long deep sleeps every night.

The medical world told me nothing was wrong with my bloodwork, even after repeating and adding more extensive panels. My next step was to visit a naturopathic thyroid clinic which used nerve testing and iodine testing to find the problem. I had a significant low functioning thyroid and was given a range of supplements to help correct things. After 4 months I had a small improvement of about 20% and so I was still searching for more support. 5 months of continuous dosing with the NES health system gave no improvement either.

Then fate stepped in – I was scrolling through a Facebook group called the Energy Medicine Exchange and came across a mention of "Biomagnetism"... Being a naturally curious wellness geek, I searched online for information about what on earth it could be! I found an American site which explained just how different it was to other therapies. And my body was in dire need of a different approach!

Further research led me to learn about a training course with Dr Goiz with English translations held in California… and the seed had been planted. The thoughts of learning this pioneering new therapy and introducing it to Australia would not let me alone… And so, a few months later I took the leap and travelled to learn the therapy by the famous Dr Goiz himself, despite never having received a session before.

I've always had strong intuition and something inside me knew this therapy would help me personally as well as my clientele in Emerald – Central Queensland.

In my first two treatments for my thyroid, all imbalances were taken care of. The fatigue that hit me at 7pm lifted completely after the second session and never returned. (7pm bedtime story time separately for three young children - Parents, you know the torture of doing this while exhausted!)

This was over ten years ago now, and in the first two years I found it highly effective for all sorts of conditions and symptoms including:

Fibromyalgia, PCOS, infertility, children's behaviours, ASD symptoms, acute infections of all types including chicken pox, influenza, H. pylori, sinusitis, appendicitis, school sores and diverticulitis.

Encouraged with so much early success, I applied myself to deeper and deeper knowledge of Biomagnetism, and it became my main modality in my practice.

One case stood out to me the most. It was confronting…

You see when I was a teenager, my otherwise healthy, fit, bright and positive Mum developed breast cancer. She caught it early, had all the surgery, radiation, chemo in a typical way. She was soon cancer free. There were a few alternative and biographical books about cancer floating around the house, but her main approach was medical. And 4-5 years later that tiny, tiny original cancer of only a few millimetres came back with a vengeance, and we lost her in only weeks.

Lisa Brough's Story

From that point onwards I sought knowledge about different treatments that weren't so toxic and unsuccessful. Cancer became a special interest.

And so, the day came in my first year as a Biomagnetism Practitioner when a late-stage cancer patient was referred to me by their doctor. Only 4 weeks left to live and very thin and depleted. I explained on the phone that Biomagnetism is not known to work for late-stage cancer, but they wanted to try in case some smaller benefits could be obtained. We performed 3 sessions in 3 days. A week after returning home I heard from the client's partner reporting the following benefits:

> *Less pain – the morphine was having more effect.*
>
> *Greatly improved mood and ability to connect with his partner and spend quality time.*
>
> *The newest growth on the stomach (visually large and bulging under the skin) had flattened and softened in only a week.*

We didn't save that man as he was too far along, but with more presence and love in his heart could make the most of his time left.

Biomagnetism Healing

This trial of fire as a practitioner strengthened me personally. I feel that even in the worst-case scenario – I could still help in some way. Biomagnetism's gentle and direct balancing effect can change the internal terrain in an immediate way – supporting the body to overcome whatever disorder or challenge it cannot correct on its own.

My love of the magnets keeps growing and I am now sharing it with Australians through providing training courses, home user's classes and conferences. No longer is it inaccessible to those outside Mexico, and the USA. More and more Australian towns and cities have caring Biomagnetism practitioners ready to help with a completely different way to support healing.

And my heart is happy ☺

Minnie's Story

I had been lucky enough to meet Rosemary on her journey of Biomagnetism therapy. I am 69 and have used many alternative modalities and am always interested in learning and feeling the different results. I am grateful for my health and actively seek to maintain it.

I met Rosemary while she was studying, so she asked me if I would like to have some sessions. I understood quickly that she was very focused on building her skills.

I watched carefully as she delivered her treatments, and I appreciated her ability to focus her energy. I have continued to watch her during several sessions, and I felt her skills and her confidence grow after each session.

She was able to articulate very clearly what she found and treated during each session, which helped me to integrate and understand how I was benefiting from each of the treatments.

Now, as before, I leave her sessions feeling more balanced and energetically heightened.

Patricia's Story

I grew up on a poultry farm with five thousand chooks for which my mother, siblings and I were responsible while Dad worked for the local council. Then, as an adult, I bred Australian native birds. At the time, this pastime gave me great pleasure.

I also recreationally smoked. That, of course wasn't a wise choice.

It took four to five years for doctors to diagnose me with 'bird-breeders lung', and in my senior years, emphysema is the result of my many years caring for birds. It was breathing in the spores present in the bird faeces that did the damage.

No doubt the smoking contributed to my ill health. I stopped smoking over twenty-five years ago, but of course, the damage was done.

A friend told me about Rosemary's therapy, so I immediately sought her help.

Before the first biomagnetism session, I was huffing and puffing walking any distance or simply walking up my sloping driveway. Even housework was difficult because of the bending. I couldn't get out of bed in the morning without bringing up significant amounts of phlegm. It was horrible. I felt horrible.

After the first biomagnetism session my daughter and a friend noted that I was coughing far less than I had been. Less in severity and in frequency. Even though I don't attend biomagnetism sessions regularly, I am still far better than I was. I experience better breathing, and I'm less puffed out with simple movement.

Work with Rosemary

Clinicians have, for four decades been using Biomagnetism and have found many conditions in a human body improve. Some resolve completely in one to three treatments while long-term illnesses require multiple sessions.

This revolutionary medical discovery is now taught at some major Universities worldwide, practiced at some hospitals and clinics and recognised by major medical institutions and governments as part of their health care programmes.[44]

As more scientists acknowledge the veracity of Biomagnetism, we can expect such treatments will lose the spurious status they have been labelled with by conventional medical professionals for so long. Magnet therapies have long been options to treat conditions and

---

[44] Global Biomagnetism Todo Los Derechos Reservados, 2021, https://globalbiomagnetism.com/about-biomagnetism accessed 25 July 2024

disorders particularly those that methods of conventional medicine don't adequately address.

Conventional medicine concentrates on treating symptoms, whereas Biomagnetism investigates the reasons behind the symptoms. Remember too, that Biomagnetism differs from magnetic therapy and magnetic acupuncture. Unlike the latter two, always be aware that Biomagnetism uses *pairs of magnets* of opposing charges to depolarise areas in the body unbalanced by pathogens.[45]

As a practitioner, I'm committed to offering Biomagnetism to all people. I want to see my clients experience as profoundly as I did the changes this natural modality is capable of; changes like those that occurred for me. With the removal of a breast and continuing Biomagnetism therapy, I am restored to health now and will endeavour to stay that way by readily availing myself of this extraordinary therapy.

---

[45]Essential Mind and Body *Biomagnetic Pair Therapy 101,* https://www.essentialmb.com/single-post/biomagnetic-pair-therapy-101 accessed 30 July 2023

Work with Rosemary

As this therapy becomes more widespread, Biomagnetism will earn its place in the care regimes of not only people with obvious illness, but those who wish to optimise their health as it presents on any stressful day.

For more information, or to book a consultation with Rosemary Walters, email her @

rosemary@biomagnetismhealing.com.au

or contact her through:

biomagnetismhealing.com.au

Rosemary is located on the north side of Brisbane.

Book your healing session today!

Acknowledgments

Rhonda Valentine Dixon – You are a gift to us all. What a wonderful experience it has been working with you throughout this project. Not only are you an amazing writer with such a gentle and delightful turn of phrase, but you are also diligent, intelligent and hard working. Your love for life and doing what you love, is inspiring for those around you, and has inspired me to pursue my love, biomagnetism, to my fullest potential. Thank you for offering to write my story and doing it so wonderfully.

If you would like Rhonda to write your story, or that of a loved one, you will find her details at the back of this book.

Lisa Brough – Thank you for your tireless efforts to increase the reach of biomagnetism throughout Australia. Your mentorship and expertise, and never-ceasing interest in studying, documenting and providing support is remarkable and graciously appreciated by the whole Australian biomagnetism community. Also, thank you for shrinking my cancer and healing me before, during and after my treatment. You probably saved my life.

Helena Guerrero – Thank you for providing my biomagnetism training. Your adherence to Dr Goiz's beliefs is very important to me, and your own Biomagnetic pair discoveries and experience continues to be invaluable.

Deborah Fay – Publishing a book had never crossed my mind, so I thank you for your patience and kindness, extreme organisation and brilliance in this field. I thoroughly enjoyed the experience with you.

Simone Feiler – Brisbane Audiobook Production. Thank you so much for stepping me through audio-recording my book. What an incredible experience. Your expertise, gentleness, openness and love was really

Acknowledgments

obvious and came through beautifully, walking me through the whole process with ease. I highly recommend your services.

Thank you for your stories:

Rachel Crossingham – Thank you for being such a wonderful practitioner and fabulous friend. To work in person with Rachel in Brisbane, please find her info at: Dandelionpatch.com.au

Lisa Pearson – You have been such a support for me as I know I have been for you. Thanks for chewing and mulling as we both gather experience and momentum in this fabulous therapy. If you'd like to work with Lisa in Toowoomba please send Rosemary Walters an email.

Rhonda, Minnie, Susan, Marlene and Patricia – Your support of me throughout my training journey and onwards and your interest in biomagnetism healing has been invaluable. I have been so grateful to see your health improvements from this fabulous therapy and hope I can continue to do so.

Further Reading

A New Treatment Method of Advanced Metastatic Tumours

https://escuelaisaacgoiz.com/2024/06/27/annals-of-clinical-case-reports/

Parasite Linked with Alzheimer's and Parkinson's Diseases, Epilepsy, and Cancer

https://www.genengnews.com/news/parasite-linked-with-alzheimers-and-parkinsons-diseases-epilepsy-and-cancer/

Surprising Alternative Therapy to Cure Long Covid: Biomagnetism

https://alivenhealthy.com/2021/11/23/surprising-alternative-therapy-to-cure-long-covid/

Biomagnetic Cancer Therapy -- Medical Biomagnetism--Biomagnetic Pair—Terrain Restoration Therapy for Cancer

https://alivenhealthy.com/2019/05/15/526/

Biomagnetic Pair Therapy and Typhoid Fever: A Pilot Study

https://pubmed.ncbi.nlm.nih.gov/29067141/

Biomagnetism Australia

Magnets, Brochures, Workshops, Business Coaching, Online Mentoring Group

https://www.biomagnetismaustralia.com

Biomagnetism Pairs UK

European Certified Training Courses. Research. Biomagnetic Pair Therapy - Goiz Biomagnetism

https://www.biomagnetismpairs.co.uk

Further Reading

Healthihub Practitioner Classified Listings

https://www.healthiihub.com/

The Bio-Magnetic Hub THE BIO-MAGNETIC HUB – A Global Resource for Everything Biomagnetism Therapy

https://www.thebiomagnetichub.com

Tatarov I, Panda A, Petkov D, Kolappaswamy K, Thompson K, Kavirayani A, Lipsky MM, Elson E, Davis CC, Martin SS, DeTolla LJ. Effect of magnetic fields on tumour growth and viability. Comp Med. 2011 Aug;61(4):339-45. PMID: 22330249; PMCID: PMC3155400.

The Tumoral Phenomenon by Dr Isaac Goiz Duran. ISBN 978-607-8451-02-9

Principles of Magnetic Therapy, Biomagnetism by Dr Richard Broeringmeyer

Biogenealogy Sourcebook by Christian Fleche ISBN 978-159477206

Emotional Patterns. Fears, Emotional States and Created Patterns by Valeria Moore. ISBN 978-1-7371275-2-9.

The Psychic Roots of Disease by Bjorn Eybl

EFFECT OF THE MEDICINAL BIOMAGNETISM TECHNIQUE ON ENDOMETRIAL POLYPS: A CASE STUDY. Lázara dos Santos Rosana et al

BIOMAGNETIC PAIR AND BIOENERGETICS APPLIED IN A REAL CASE OF CERVICAL AND PANCREATIC CANCER. Silvia Joachim Rodriguez.

Further Reading

MEDICINAL BIOMAGNETISMO IN THE TREATMENT OF PROSTATE CANCER: A CASE STUDY. Angela Mara Rambo Martini, Luciane Neris Cazella, Yuri Martini, Adriane Viapiana Bossa, Jefferson Souza Santos. ISSN: 2763-5724 Vol. 03 - n 01 - ano 2023 Editora Acadêmica Periodicojs. Brazil.

TREATING PROSTATE ADENOCARCINOMA WITH BIOMAGNETISM. David Goiz Martínez and Mario Salinas Soto

Treatment of Chronic Myeloid Leukemia by Means of Medical Biomagnetism and Medical Bioenergetics.

A note from Rhonda Valentine Dixon

It was during a conversation over the fence that I realised Rosemary needed to market herself and her practice.

"Why don't I write your story?" I said to her.

I'd had some sessions with Rosemary myself. I believed every human would benefit from this extraordinary therapy because it's as much preventative as it is restorative.

This book is the result of that chat over the fence.

Rosemary has been a delight to work with.

I'm honoured to have been a part of highlighting Rosemary and her Biomagnetism practice.

Rhonda the Writer

For me, completing a BA (Hons) in Literary Studies was a step towards becoming a writer. However, achieving the University of Tasmania's Diploma of Family History gave me the direction I wanted to take. Telling people's stories.

My Creative Biography includes:

- Co-authoring three books to assist autistic children and their families

- Publishing articles relating to the Autism Spectrum and the NDIS

- Independently publishing a children's picture book

- Publishing articles in two 'what's on in our region' magazines.

Author Achievements include

- Four times long listed in an international competition

- Short listed in a Queensland competition

- Two Honourable Mentions in an international competition.

A note from Rhonda Valentine Dixon

Professional Organisations

Queensland Writers' Centre

You can contact me at rtvdixon@gmail.com or www.rhondavalentinedixon.com.au

If you, as a friend or client of Rosemary, need your story written, please don't hesitate to get in touch with me. I'd be happy to discuss writing your story with you.

www.ingramcontent.com/pod-product-compliance
Lightning Source LLC
Chambersburg PA
CBHW061738070526
44585CB00024B/2723